A MAXWELL WINSTON STONE SERIES

# Attitude

## It's Not *What* You See,
## It's *How* You See

## ERNIE CARWILE

1

A MAXWELL WINSTON STONE SERIES

# Attitude

## It's Not *What* You See,
## It's *How* You See

## ERNIE CARWILE

**Verbena Pond Publishing Co., L.L.C.**

www.VerbenaPondPublishing.com.
Email: erniecarwile@comcast.net

2012 2011 2010 2009

ISBN: 978-0-9796176-3-8

Library of Congress Control Number:    2007941998

Printed in Canada

*This book is dedicated to the truth that lies within each of us which knows that our attitude drastically affects everything we experience in life.*

## OTHER BOOKS BY ERNIE CARWILE

THE MAX CHRONICLES presents *THE STORYTELLER 1*

*CHIPPED BUT NOT BROKEN: When Adversity Enhances the Human Spirit*

*NEVER GOOD ENOUGH: Discover the Treasure of Self-Acceptance*

*WHERE DO WE GO FROM HERE? Death, the Next Great Adventure*

*PERSISTENCE: The Art of Failing Until You Succeed*

*RECLAIMING THE POWER OF SILENCE*

*CONNECTED BY THE SOUL: Oh, The Oneness of Us all*

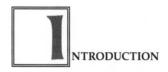

# INTRODUCTION

This is the seventh book in THE MAXWELL WINSTON STONE SERIES. Like the others, this topic disclosed itself one day while I was reading *another* book of quotes. Suddenly, as if the clouds temporarily parted, I was able to see that there were recurrent themes being written by the wisest of each generation throughout all of history. After reviewing many, many quotes going back twenty-five hundred years to the time of Plato and Socrates, I was able to identify fifteen of these recurring themes that we humans have repeatedly experienced.

Then an insightful question popped into my head: If solutions to life's problems had been discovered and used by the wisest from each generation before us, then why couldn't *everyone* on our planet have the opportunity to benefit from this great wisdom? Thus, my journey of writing on these fifteen, precious, recurring themes began.

This seventh book is on *Attitude* and its power in affecting our lives is of such a powerful magnitude that we are only beginning to understand its vastness and implications because of recent discoveries from quantum physics.

*** 

Early in my life, burned into my memories, were the efforts of coaches and teachers etching the old adage that my attitude strongly affects everything I will experience. Over and over, I heard, like a set-in-concrete, high-amplified, broken phonograph, the phrase *Attitude Is Everything* being retold continuously throughout my life.

However, until the recent finding of *quantum physics*, I did not fully comprehend just how encompassing and powerful one's attitude reflects in one's perception. Why? Because quantum physics, for the first time in the history of our world, actually brought us scientific proof that when we observe something, the act of observation changes the *reality* of that object.

Quantum physics …

Just the word itself intimidates me, leaving me with feelings of inadequacy—my inability to keep up with the prodigious number of new scientific discoveries bombarding our world today.

But, just for a moment, I urge us to let loose of the overwhelmingness of all these new ideas and simply focus on just one, new single insight that the science of quantum physics has bestowed upon us: *As we observe an object, we change the make-up of that object.*

By the way, this new truth is to be taken literally. Repeat: we actually change an object when we look at it.

Once this concept enters into your consciousness and you come to grasp its significance, your understanding of the topic of *attitude* will revolutionize your life. Remember that the wisest of each generation in our world's history have been attempting to remind us all of the power of attitude, now we understand just why they have done so. Have a negative attitude, and the world becomes bleak, dark and hopeless. Have a positive outlook and the world will suddenly, as if by magic, portray a bright, opportunistic and kinder place in which you live.

We have all heard the much-used, positive think-ing lesson about the infamous glass of water: Is it half full or half empty?

Now with this new piece of information, the mean-ing behind this little ditty takes on gargantuan propor-tions. Bursting forth in new freshness we realize that *how we see is more important that what we see*—that how we observe something actually changes it—that each of our attitudes about everything we encounter in our lives creates the kind of reality we will experience.

Or, as the wise old philosopher Maxwell Winston Stone said, "It is truly a spectacular awakening when you finally realize it is only you who is limiting yourself."

Now sit back, relax, *remember* and enjoy.

Ernie Carwile

Note: It is easier to observe attitudes in other people than yourself. However, there are two sound ways for you to discover who you are. One, look at the things in your life, the good and the bad. They are proof of what kind of attitude you are projecting. Second, ask a good friend to help you see how you come across to the world. Then evaluate and decide if you wish to change.

Attitude is a little thing that makes a big difference.

—WINSTON CHURCHILL
(1874–1965)

**I**F YOU HAVE NOT READ any of the prior books in THE MAXWELL WINSTON STONE SERIES, you may wish to start with the first book, *CHIPPED BUT NOT BROKEN: When Adversity Enhances The Human Spirit*, then follow with the others. In doing this, you will learn more about my friend, Max. But for now, suffice it to say he was someone who monumentally affected my life through a seemingly unending storehouse of stories and quotes which were all applicable to the life difficulties I was experiencing. Never preachy, Max just had a knack for speaking simply and frankly to problems we humans get to deal with.

Today was another of those days. He just started up out of the blue—no preamble or anything.

"Okay Ernie, let me try to make this as clear and simple as possible."

Not knowing what he was even talking about, I said, "Sure."

"Now we've all heard that a good attitude is important in life ... right?"

"Yep," I agreed, but inwardly thought that this little learning session wasn't going to be very profound, nor anything new.

"Stay with me now," Max said while reading my facial expression. "I know you, and I can see you're probably thinking this is too simplistic."

I grinned, knowing that my friend knew me all too well, and then said, "Guilty as charged."

Max paused and I sensed his brain was churning. "You have inside you a perceiver, you know, a person who sees something; and you have an object or event—outside you—which the perceiver views.

"Now the mood, or frame of reference, or mind-set of the perceiver *colors* everything that he or she looks at."

Max leaned toward me for emphasis, "Forget the object or event. It's what is going on in the perceiver's mind which is the crux of everything."

"But what about the object or event, Max? Doesn't it have anything to do with what a person sees?"

"Good questions, Ernie. But this is what I want you to really understand and get … The actual object or event being observed is no where near as important as the mindset of the perceiver. If the perceiver is angry, or sad, afraid or whatever, that emotion greatly affects everything the person sees and reacts to."

I found myself a bit perplexed. Whereas on one hand I thought I already knew what Max had just explained; on the other hand his explanation made my understanding immensely better … I mean, I knew my mind-set certainly affected whatever I was doing, but I had just never understood the magnitude with which it colored my whole life.

"You never cease to amaze me, Max," I said while shaking my head in awe.

Max grinned like the cheshire cat.

Happiness is a choice. It is something you decide on ahead of time ... It's how you *arrange* your thoughts that counts.

—MAXWELL WINSTON STONE

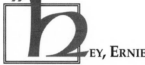"Hey, Ernie," Max was smiling. "I've got a story for you."

"A story … now that's a real shocker," I replied, ribbing my friend over his seemingly never-ending supply of stories he has stored away.

Still grinning, Max proceeded, "I heard about an eighty-eight-year-old man. He arose each morning by seven-thirty; shaved, combed his fashionably cut hair and donned a white shirt and tie. Every single day he did this, despite the fact that he was legally blind.

"His wife had recently died, making it necessary for him to make the move to a nursing home and leave their home of sixty some years.

"Arriving at the home, he was told his room was not quite ready and he would have to wait. After waiting a long while, he was finally escorted to an elevator where the nurse began describing his tiny little room and where everything had been placed.

"'I love it, already,' he happily proclaimed.

"'But you haven't even seen it yet,' she retorted with a small grin.

"'That has nothing to do with it,' he matter-of-factly said, 'happiness is something you decide upon ahead of time. Whether or not I like my room has little to do with the room and furniture itself. What counts is how I arrange my thoughts, and I've already decided I love it.'

"The young nurse was in awe of the words and wisdom this little, old man was sharing.

"He continued, 'It's a decision I make every morning when I wake up. I have a choice; I can lay there in bed focusing on all the parts of my body that don't work anymore, or I can get up and give thanks for the ones that still do.'

"'I have come to see that each day is a gift,' he explained, 'and that each day when I awaken I'll focus on all the happy memories in my life that I've stored away for just this moment.'

"Pausing, he added, 'I believe old age is kind of like a bank account where you can withdraw from the savings you've put into it.'"

Max finished the story saying, "I like that old man's attitude."

"Me too, Max," I nodded, "me too."

We don't see things
as they are; we see
things as we are.

—ANAIS NIN, AUTHOR
(1914–1977)

**D**O YOU REMEMBER who invented the first steamboat? Think back to when you were in school, if you can recall that far back. It was Robert Fulton.

What you may not know was what actually took place at the first test run of the ship named, *The Clermont*. A crowd had gathered on the shore and watched as this strange, new ship built up steam and spewed and shot out sparks from its tall, thin smoke stacks.

Extremely pessimistic and negative towards the new invention, the people suddenly broke out in unison, "She'll never start! She'll never start!"

But of course, as we all know, she did start and successfully moved up the river.

Here's what is so important to remember. Do you know what that negative group then started shouting after recovering from their amazement? … "She'll never stop! She'll never stop!"

The best thing you could say about those people, I guess is that they had, at least, a consistently negative attitude.

Attitude is everything
in life. Some complain
that roses have thorns,
while others give thanks
that thorns have roses.

—MAXWELL WINSTON STONE

*T*HERE WAS A SEASONED salesman who was sent by his company to Africa to open up a new market. His company was a shoe manufacturer; they had retail outlets all over the world, but had never tried the African market.

They were very anxious to see if this could be a promising market and wanted to hear from their representative quite badly. A week passed by … then two. Of course, by now they had become worried about him. Had he been hurt? Had he even arrived?

Finally, after four weeks they received a cablegram saying, "Coming home on the next plane. Situation just hopeless. No one here wears shoes!"

The company was quite disappointed since they had high expectations for the new market. After much discussion, they finally decided to send over a relatively new salesman to try one more time. Again they waited.

Just like before they heard nothing from him for one week … then two … then three. At the beginning of the fourth week they finally received a cablegram, but this time the message read: "Having the time of my life. Over 1,000 orders have been mailed to you. This place is incredible. The opportunities are limitless. You see, no one wears shoes here!"

We have the choice to either make ourselves miserable and weak, or happy and strong. What is so interesting is that it takes the *same amount* of energy to achieve either.

—Maxwell Winston Stone

## The Way You Look at Things

Attitude reigns all,
    more real than a rock.
It colors the world we see,
    As tight as any knot.

In the blink of an eye,
    a judgment is made.
Like a clamp of a jaw,
    our minds become set.

In only a second,
    that's all it took.
We hope it is sound,
    Like the world proved round.

Right or wrong is indifferent,
    for it is only our take.
God help us if we're wrong,
    for in life there is no remake.

Particles not touching,
    We've learned there is no firmament,
Only our attitude,
    is exactly what we get.

—ERNIE CARWILE

If you're in a hole;
stop digging.

—MAXWELL WINSTON STONE

*T*WO MEN WHO WORKED on a highrise office building ate lunch together every day at noon. Each day, as the men opened up their lunch boxes, one of the men always complained about having to eat the same miserable thing—a cheese sandwich.

This same event occurred every day, and every day the other man had to hear the rantings and ravings over the one's dislike of cheese sandwiches.

Finally, becoming completely fed up over hearing the same complaint day in and day out, the other man screamed, "Well, who makes your lunch?"

To which the guy took a bite out of his cheese sandwich and calmly replied, "Oh, I do!"

People are affected not
by things, but by the views
they take on those things.

—MAXWELL WINSTON STONE

"HEY ERNIE, did you know in criminal trials, an eyewitness identifying the accused is one of the most unreliable testimony for the prosecutor?"

"How is that Max," I said surprisingly asked.

"Because any good defense attorney knows that if three people view an incident, there is almost never just one version of what happens, but often times there are three different stories."

"Why, Max?" He had my interest now.

"Because whenever a person sees something, they are seeing through filters—or *glasses made from their past experiences and their current state of mind.* For example, if you have a witness to a rape who had also been a rape victim herself, let's say by a tall bearded man, and that witness saw some *tall bearded man* near the scene of the crime, let me tell you," Max sadly shook his head, "that other man, even if he is totally innocent, is in big trouble.

"All of us see through these filters or glasses which represent a *bent* or an attitude which colors everything we see. Thus the subtitle of this book, *IT'S HOW YOU SEE, NOT WHAT YOU SEE THAT COUNTS.*"

"Max," I said, "You are a most interesting fellow."

No one can control
life; only their
response to it.

—MAXWELL WINSTON STONE

Just remember that a plumber and Michelangelo the painter got their marble from the same quarry.

The difference is that one saw a nobleman's toilet or sink ... while the other saw a magnificent sculpture.

—MAXWELL WINSTON STONE

Just one person with a strong attitude is better than a hundred with only a minor interest.

—MAXWELL WINSTON STONE

**M**AX AND **I** WERE driving back to his house after doing volunteer work at one of the homeless shelters in Denver. We would always discuss the men we had come into contact with—their problems, usually mental as well as addictions, and their seemingly hopeless lives. Every once in a while, though, we would talk with one whose attitude singularly set them apart from all the others. We met a man like that tonight and both of us sensed and hoped for the possibilities of a life changing direction, something we rarely saw. Unlike many of the others who seemed too ready to volunteer their dire life situations, Reuben was very different. In fact, we had to repeatedly coax him to open up to us. And once he did, his story proved tortuous to hear. Yet, there remained a stillness and attitude within his words that emitted a small aura of light.

"Maybe Reuben will be able to turn his life around," Max stated.

"I hope so," I said, "he certainly possesses a different frame of mind than most of the men."

Max cleared his throat before speaking. "One of the most phenomenal stories on attitude I have ever heard was about a polio victim named Karl Sudekum. Although he was completely paralyzed in his body just below his Adam's apple, he eventually did the impossible by leaving his iron lung and learning to breath like a frog."

I took my eyes off the road for just a second, turned to look at Max and said, "You gotta be kidding me."

"Nope," Max continued, "while a lieutenant in the Navy in 1953, he contracted polio. For six long years, the only way he could breathe was in an iron lung, on a tilt bed. His life seemed hopeless until one day he got really angry and decided he would find another way to breathe—outside his metal prison.

"Searching his memories, he suddenly remembered how he used to breathe like a frog as a young boy. You probably remember the trick," Max said. "It's where you take in a gulp of air and then force it down your windpipe.

My head was nodding up and down. "Of course," I said.

"And when he exhaled, his lungs let out the air like a deflating balloon …" Max laughed, "He's been breathing that way ever since … and science doesn't know how it's done."

I grinned with sheer appreciation.

"The guy said it's like whistling through your teeth; some people can do it and some can't."

"Wow," I sighed.

"His next decision was to become an attorney, so he entered the University of San Diego where his wife drove him to school and wheeled him into class. He couldn't take notes and a tape recorder was too cumbersome. His solution? … He learned to listen and remember very well."

Max continued, "Other problems entered this amazing man's life, like developing diabetes and an ulcer. But he eventually got his diploma and passed California's bar exam."

All I could do was shake my head in wonderment.

"He began practicing law and signed his name 'K.D. Sudekum' by writing with a pen in his teeth.

"When he talked too long in court, his face became red, though he learned to handle it. But the big problem involved getting a cold, something that could easily prove fatal … so what did he do?" Max glowed.

"Sudekum boldly stated, 'I don't get colds.'

"If he falls asleep or faints outside the iron lungs doing his frog breathing, he will die … what does he do about that? He said, 'I try to think about it as little as possible!'"

"Gee Max," I said, "now this is a guy with an attitude I wish I could have."

"Oh you can, Ernie," Max affirmed with utmost sincerity, "you most certainly can."

Oh, my friend, it's not what they take from you that counts. It's what you do with what you have left.

—HUBERT A. HUMPHREY
(1911–1978)

An optimist is someone
who believes we live in
the best possible world.
The pessimist is afraid
that this is true.

—MAXWELL WINSTON STONE

**I**T DOESN'T TAKE AGE OR MATURITY to develop a good attitude. It's so simple even a child can have it.

A Sunday school teacher had been closely watching one of her kindergarten students. More than any of the other kids, he was especially straining and grimacing to get whatever he was drawing just right.

Unable to control her curiosity, she finally walked over to the little boy and asked, "What are you drawing Billy?"

Billy replied, "A picture of God."

Astounded, the teacher gasped, "But, Billy, no one knows what God looks like."

Smiling confidently, Billy said, "They will after I'm finished!"

Whether you believe
you can do a thing, or
not do it, you are right.

—HENRY FORD
(1863–1947)

"**O**FTEN TIMES, A SMALL CHANGE IN attitude will make a huge change in someone's life," Max proclaimed.

"Hey Max, I know that," I replied, a bit taken back.

"Well, I bet you haven't heard this next story."

With only a hint of a smile, he began.

"I once heard about a small boy who lived in Italy and absolutely loved music. The only problem with this was that he had no musical talent. I mean he couldn't sing a lick, nor could he play any instrument even though he had tried and tried.

"Frustrated, he shared his predicament about not being able to contribute something musical to the world with a friend—an old man named Amati who made violins.

"Now this old man could have dismissed this little boy's dreams, but instead he gave him the most important gifts of hope and encouragement. He told the boy that the song in one's heart is all that matters and that there were many ways to make music—some play, some sing, some paint pictures, some create beautiful sculptures and some grow wonderful flowers.

"He assured the boy, 'You too, can make music.'

"The little boy returned home with a new attitude about his abilities now that a whole new world of opportunities had suddenly opened up to him.

"Many years later, that little boy who had no talent to either sing, or play any instrument well, made one of the greatest contributions to the world in music. How? By becoming the greatest violin maker of all time.

"Of course, his name was Antonio Stradivarius."

Like always, I could only stand in amazement at Max's story.

There is neither good
nor bad, but thinking
that makes it so.

—WILLIAM SHAKESPEARE
(1564–1616)

To everyone is given the key to heaven; The same key opens the gates to hell.

—ANCIENT PROVERB

*A* YOUNG MAN JOINED a very strict monastery where talking was forbidden.

There was one exception to this rule of silence: once every three years, each monk could meet with the abbot and express one thing that had been on his mind the past years. However, the rule dictated that each monk could only speak three words.

After the first three years, the monk sat down with the abbot and said, "food is bad," after which he returned to his cell.

Three years later he again met with the abbot and this time said, "bed too hard."

After the next three years had elapsed, he met with his abbot and said, "Want to leave."

The crusty old abbot stared at the man for quite a while before saying, "It doesn't surprise me. You've complained the whole time you were here."

What you *think* is
what you *feel.*

—MAXWELL WINSTON STONE

*T*WO COMPLETE STRANGERS met on a path in the woods. Going to the same destination, they decided to travel together.

One of the men believed the path led to a great wondrous place; the other believed it led to no place special.

During their journey, they encountered both difficulties and pleasant times. All the while, one's attitude perceived the journey to be an almost holy expedition. He saw obstacles as tests of his commitment and pleasant surprises as blessings of encouragement.

The other continued with his bleak attitude, and experienced the whole trip as nothing more than a difficult, meaningless journey.

When they arrived at their journey, do you know what each discovered?

They were both right!

Each person is the
sculptor and director
of their own life.

—MAXWELL WINSTON STONE

*a* MANAGER OF A LARGE STORE had a talk with his employees, emphasizing to them the importance of their attitudes when dealing with the customers. He encouraged them to always give their best effort and shared an analogy to help them better understand what he was saying.

"Thousands of years ago," he began, "a gargantuan building project began using slaves. He described to them three particular slaves who were representative of all the workers working there. He said the viewpoint that each of these three slaves had toward their job differed greatly.

"One saw his job as nothing more than the arduous tasks of cutting out the rock and dragging it back to the building site.

"Another viewed his job as one of building a wall.

"While the third viewed his job as if he were creating a beautiful church.

"Each did the same thing and each worked hard every day."

And then the manager asked these powerful, powerful questions: "Which one do you think looked forward to the next day's work? And, which one would you want to work next to?"

If you look for beauty,
you'll find it.
Look for imperfections,
you'll find them too.

—MAXWELL WINSTON STONE

"ERNIE," MAX SAID, "I want to share a legend with you. It may seem simple and obvious at first, but I want to see if you can grasp its power."

"Okay," I said, "fire away."

"A long, long time ago in a kingdom far, far away ruled a very wise queen. One day she called two of her greatest knights together and gave each one separate instructions.

"To one she instructed that he travel throughout her kingdom and bring back samples of *only* poisonous plants. To the other the instructions were to look for and bring back samples of *only* the most beautiful plants. She strongly emphasized that each was to follow her exact instructions.

"Upon returning, a most interesting, though seemingly simplistic fact emerged: each knight had returned with only the plants they had focused on. The knight, who had sought beautiful flowers, brought only samples of beautiful flowers. The knight who only looked for poisonous plants, returned with only samples of those."

Max leaned close to me and with great emphasis asked, "Do you see? Vision is of the mind—our attitude is like a pair of eyeglasses. We seek only that which we are seeking and we receive only that which we have been looking for."

Shaking my head in astonishment, I slowly said, "You have done it again, Max."

"See, it's just like us, only there's no queen instructing what to seek and to find. *We* are the ones who do that to ourselves. If you want to see the type of attitude you carry around, look at the things that you have. They will disclose what you have been focusing upon."

"Max, trust me on this one. I get it."

People are just as
happy as they make up
their minds to be.

—ABRAHAM LINCOLN
(1809–1865)

**S**OMETIMES, IF WE ARE LUCKY, our attitude will be reflected back to us so we can see how foolish we've been.

In the early 1900's, a bishop was invited to meet with a college president and the faculty of the physics department.

During this meeting, the president asked the learned bishop what he believed would be the next major advancements in technology, especially in the area of humans learning to fly.

Very arrogantly the bishop retorted, "Man will never fly. Why, if God wanted us to fly, He would have given us wings."

The missing element in this story is that the bishop was from Dayton, Ohio and his last name was W-R-I-G-H-T. Even more intriguing is that in only a few short years, it would be his own two sons, Wilbur

and Orville, who would be the first persons to fly an
airplane at Kitty Hawk …

It isn't our *position* but our *disposition* that makes us happy.

—MAXWELL WINSTON STONE

*a* VERY WEALTHY FATHER wanted to teach his son appreciation for what he had by showing him how poor people lived. So after many telephone calls he arranged for them both to spend two days and nights on a farm most people would consider rather paltry.

Driving home with his son after the two days, the father asked him the pertinent question, "Did you see how poor people live?"

"You bet, I did," the boy replied.

"Well, what did you learn?" the father further questioned.

After a brief moment in collecting his thoughts, the boy responded;

"I saw that we buy our food, but they grow theirs ... and theirs tastes better.

"I saw they had four dogs where we only have one.

"We have only a small piece of land and they have acres and acres.

"We have a backyard swimming pool that is tiny compared to their creek.

"We have walls surrounding our property. They have friends to protect them.

"We have servants who serve us; they serve others."

The boy's father was stunned—dumbfounded.

Then the boy concluded, "Thanks for showing me how poor we are, Dad."

Attitude can be a wonderful thing, can't it?

Weakness of attitude
becomes weakness
of character.

—ALBERT EINSTEIN
(1879–1955)

"We've been talking and reading a lot about how attitude affects how and what a person actually sees. There may be many aspects that a person might view, and it is their attitudes which defines what they see," Max said.

"Yes, yes, yes, Max, I understand this."

"I heard of a man that purchased an experienced black Labrador and was anxious to try the new dog out to see how well it retrieved.

"The next morning, standing next to his dog in a duck blind, some ducks flew over and the man shot one down. As soon as the duck hit the water the man watched as the dog skipped out on the water, tiptoed over, picked up the duck and returned without ever getting wet.

"I couldn't have seen what I just saw," the man whispered to himself.

"But again, as new ducks flew over he shot one, and, sure enough, the dog skimmed out onto the water, tiptoed over to the fallen duck, picked it up and returned without getting a drop of water on himself.

"A friend of the man was in the blind next to him. Still amazed, he took his dog over to the other man's blind and said, 'Bob, watch this.'

"When more ducks flew over, this time the man shot down another duck and both men watched as the dog skipped out onto the water, picked up the fallen duck, then tiptoed back to the hunters dry as a bone.

"The man with the amazing dog said to his friend, Bob, 'How about that? Did you see anything remarkable about what my dog just did?'

"'Sure,' Bob said matter-of-factly, 'your dog can't swim!'"

As I burst out laughing, Max concluded his story by saying, "See what I mean. It all depends on how you look at something."

I think life is like a
boomerang. Everything we
say and do comes back to
us with exact accuracy.

—MAXWELL WINSTON STONE

JUST FOR A
MOMENT, CLOSE
YOUR EYES
AND RECALL
THE ATTITUDE
YOU HAD WHEN
INTERACTING
WITH THE PEOPLE
WITH WHOM
YOU CAME INTO
CONTACT TODAY ...

You are *only* responsible
for your own reactions
to life situations.

—MAXWELL WINSTON STONE

The mind is its own place, and in itself can make a Heav'n of Hell, a Hell of Heav'n.

—JOHN MILTON
(1608–1674)

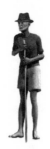

*T*HERE ONCE WAS A MAN who had an obsession that he was dead. Finally, his friends convinced him to visit a psychiatrist for help.

The very successful psychiatrist tried all of the known techniques and tools to help the man see that he was alive, but none worked.

Finally, the psychiatrist decided to appeal to good, old-fashioned logic. "Do dead men bleed?" asked the doctor.

"No, no, of course not," the patient replied.

"All right then," said the doctor, "let's try an experiment."

Taking a sharp needle the doctor pricked the man's skin and the wound began to bleed.

"See!" exclaimed the psychiatrist, "What do you say now?"

"Well, I'll be darned!" responded the patient in astonishment, "Dead people do bleed!"

The mind is everything;
what you think, you become.

—BUDDHA

**I** HEARD ABOUT A STUDY that was conducted on the effects of alcoholism on young children. Two of the subjects were twin brothers who had been raised by an alcoholic father. When they achieved adulthood, each chose to move away from their home environment and live in different parts of the country.

Years later they were re-interviewed by the same psychiatrist who had been conducting the research. He made a startling discovery. What he found was that these two men reared in the same exact home ended up as radically different people.

One became a doctor, a pillar of his community; was creative and hopeful about life. The other became bitter and angry.

When interviewing the bitter and angry young man in prison and learning how he had developed his outlook on life, the man replied, *"What else would you have expected if you had grown up with a father like mine."*

The psychiatrist later interviewed the positive and hopeful brother and posed the same question. His response proved to be greatly surprising and one we all should never forget. He too, said, *"What else would you expect if you had a father like mine,"* the exact same words his brother in prison had used.

For as he thinketh
in his heart,
so is he.

—PROVERBS 23:7
KING JAMES VERSION

## Willie Duncan's Story

**I** BELONG TO THE Greenwood Athletic and Tennis Club, just abutting Denver, Colorado. After joining, I kept running into a man named Willie Duncan, who worked in the men's locker room. What was so impressive about him was his ever uplifting disposition, as well as phenomenal memory for members' names. Every visit, I would either observe or hear him fondly greeting each member by their name, and often even their family member's names. His concern and interest in everyone was genuine, and this genuineness was simply infectious. Truly, his interactions with people enhanced everyone's daily lives.

One day, as I was just finishing using the urinal, I happened to look down on the floor and saw an inordinate amount of droppings by others who obviously had some severely deficient aiming skills. At that same moment Willie entered the bathroom carrying supplies and I heard his upbeat greeting, "Good morning, Ernie." To which I replied over my shoulder, "Willie, unfortunately for you too many men seem to have splattered all over the floor."

Now, this was his response, stated with no delay whatsoever, "I look at that, Ernie, as job security!"

Only after I stopped laughing did this rare man's fantastic attitude clearly materialize for me. Many months later when I reminded him of his uniquely wonderful response, with a most serious demeanor, he replied, "Ernie, every day I can choose to either be mad and sorry for my life ... or, I can be positive and joyful about it."

Just then a quote by Mark Twain popped into my head, "I never met a man from whom I couldn't learn something" ... and Mr. Willie Duncan, a treasure of the Greenwood Athletic and Tennis Club, strengthens the validity of that sage advice and provides a power-ful role model for me to try and emulate.

Ernie Carwile

It is something to be
able to paint a picture,
or to carve a statue—to
make a few objects
beautiful. But it is far
more glamorous to
carve and paint *the very
atmosphere and medium*
through which we look.

—HENRY DAVID THOREAU
**(1817–1862)**

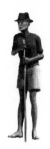

"**I**T SEEMS THAT THERE will always be negative people around. You know who I mean—people who just try to bring us down.

"When you run into one of them, remember this story."

A woman had started going to a new hairdresser. She didn't particularly like the lady, was looking for a replacement, but for now was stuck with her. She happened to mention to the hair dresser that she and her husband were going on a dream vacation to Rome.

The hairdresser responded, "Rome. Why in the world would anyone visit there? There are pickpockets galore. Its dirty … How are you getting there?"

"We're taking United Airlines," the lady replied, "We got a great rate."

"United," the hairdresser smugly said, "they are the worst airline around. The flight attendants are rude, their planes are old and they're always late ... Where are you staying in Rome?"

With a bit of hesitation now, the lady replied, "We'll be at a very exclusive place on the Tiber River."

"You're kidding me. I've heard of that place," the hairdresser moaned. "It's really a dump. The rooms are small, service is rotten and it's way overpriced ... What are you going to do when you get there?"

"We're going to the Vatican, and ... we hope to see the Pope," the now embarrassed lady sheepishly replied.

"Ha," said the hairdresser, "you and a million other suckers. You'll be so far back the Pope will look like the size of an ant."

Distressed, the woman paid and then left.

However, a month later, she returned to the same hairdresser armed with wonderful news. When the hairdresser asked about her trip, she began.

"Fantastic," the woman said, "when we arrived at United, they were overbooked and bumped us up to business class. The food, wine and service were just impeccable ... and the hotel was gorgeous. They'd just finished a seven million dollar remodeling job and it is truly the best of Italy."

"Well, "muttered the hairdresser, "That may be, but I know you didn't get to see the Pope," she defiantly pressed.

"Actually, something quite extraordinary happened. While we were touring the Vatican one of the Swiss guards approached us, explained the Pope liked to meet some of the visitors in private and invited us in to meet him. Believe it or not, we were soon escorted in and the Pope walked up and shook my hand."

The hairdresser stood transfixed.

"When I knelt down to kiss his ring, the Pope leaned down and spoke a few words to me."

"What did he say?" the hairdresser astoundedly asked.

"He said: 'Who cuts your hair? You got a really lousy haircut.'"

It's easy to recognize
the people who have
good attitudes—they
are usually *smiling*.

—MAXWELL WINSTON STONE

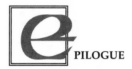 **PILOGUE**

We just recently made a rather amazing discovery. Our son, Cole, lives in Alaska. One evening while a friend was visiting him, the young man shared that he was dealing with a problem, something males unfortunately seldom share with other males.

Cole, unsure of what advice to give, picked up a copy of my first book in THE MAXWELL WINSTON STONE SERIES, *CHIPPED BUT NOT BROKEN: When Adversity Enhances The Human Spirit,* and tossed the book to his friend. He then told him to open the book to any page and declared that the solution to his problem would be shown to him.

His friend did so, read the page he had opened, then suddenly tossed the book back to Cole with a yelp. He proclaimed, "How in the world did you know that would work?"

After this, we began experimenting with all of the books in this series and each time it proved true.

Therefore, you also might experiment. Simply choose a book that relates to a current problem you are experiencing. Then open the book to any place and within a few moments, see if you don't receive an answer … It's amazing.

THE MAXWELL WINSTON STONE SERIES … Solutions to Life's problems.

Our world is filled with people who hold a "poor me," victim-consciousness ... fortunately, many are beginning to realize it is their very own mind-set which brings about what they experience in life.

—Maxwell Winston Stone

# A Great Gift Idea!

(Share the gift of these books with others)

**To Purchase:**

| | | |
|---|---|---|
| 1. | *Attitude* | $10.00 +<br>$1.00 Shipping per book |
| 2. | *Connected By the Soul* | $12.00 +<br>$1.00 Shipping per book |
| 3. | *Reclaiming the Power of Silence* | $10.00 +<br>$1.00 Shipping per book |
| 4. | *Persistence* | $10.00 +<br>$1.00 Shipping per book |
| 5. | *Where Do We Go From Here* | $10.00 +<br>$1.00 Shipping per book |
| 6. | *Never Good Enough* | $10.00 +<br>$1.00 Shipping per book |
| 7. | *Chipped But Not Broken* | $10.00+<br>$1.00 Shipping per book |
| 8. | *The Storyteller 1* | $14.95+<br>$1.00 Shipping per book |

Quality discounts available. Call Ernie at 303-641-8632

## THREE WAYS TO ORDER:

**1. Send a check to:**

    **OR**

Verbena Pond Publishing
P.O. Box 370270
Denver, CO 80237

**2. PayPal on our website**

*www.MaxwellWinstonStone.com*

**3. Order through**

*Amazon.com*

## RECOMMENDED READING

*CONNECTED BY THE SOUL: Oh, The Oneness Of Us All*, Ernie Carwile. Verbena Pond Publishing, P.O. Box 370270, Denver, CO 80237. $12.00 U.S. plus $1.00 shipping each book. *www.MaxwellWinstonStone.com* or order at *www.Amazon.com.*

*RECLAIMING THE POWER OF SILENCE*, Ernie Carwile. Verbena Pond Publishing, P.O. Box 370270, Denver, CO 80237. $10.00 U.S. plus $1.00 shipping each book. *www.MaxwellWinstonStone.com* or order at *www.Amazon.com.*

*PERSISTENCE: The Art of Failing Until You Succeed*, Ernie Carwile. Verbena Pond Publishing, P.O. Box 370270, Denver, CO 80237. $10.00 U.S. plus $1.00 shipping each book. *www.MaxwellWinstonStone.com* or order at *www.Amazon.com.*

*WHERE DO WE GO FROM HERE? Death, The Next Great Adventure*, Ernie Carwile. Verbena Pond Publishing, P.O. Box 370270, Denver, CO 80237. $10.00 U.S. plus $1.00 shipping each book. *www.MaxwellWinstonStone.com* or order at *www.Amazon.com.*

**NEVER GOOD ENOUGH:** *Discover the Treasure of Self-Acceptance*, Ernie Carwile. Verbena Pond Publishing, P.O. Box 370270, Denver, CO 80237. $10.00 U.S. plus $1.00 shipping each book. *www.MaxwellWinstonStone.com* or order at *www.Amazon.com.*

**CHIPPED BUT NOT BROKEN:** *When Adversity Enhances The Human Spirit*, Ernie Carwile. Verbena Pond Publishing, P.O. Box 370270, Denver, CO 80237. $10.00 U.S. plus $1.00 shipping each book. *www.ChippedButNotBroken.com* or order at *www.Amazon.com.*

**THE MAX CHRONICLES** *presents THE STORYTELLER 1*, Ernie Carwile. Verbena Pond Publishing, P.O. Box 370270, Denver, CO 80237. $14.95 plus $1.00 shipping each book. *www.MaxwellWinstonStone.com* or order at *www.Amazon.com.*

**HEART STRINGS AT 35,000 FEET,** Mary Catherine Carwile. Verbena Pond Publishing, P.O. Box 370270, Denver, CO 80237. $12.95 plus $1.00 shipping each book. *www.MaryCarwile.com* or order at *www.Amazon.com.*

*HEARTSTRINGS AND PINK RIBBONS: Finding Comfort Until There's A Cure,* Mary Catherine Carwile. Verbena Pond Publishing, P.O. Box 370270, Denver, CO 80237. $15.00 plus $2.00 shipping each book. *www.MaryCarwile.com* or order at *www.Amazon.com.*

*TO BEE or NOT TO BEE: A Book for Beings Who Feel There's More To Life Than Just Making Honey,* John Penberthy. *www.ToBeeBook.com.*

*ONENESS: By Rasha.* Earthstar Press, 369 Montezuma Ave. #321, Santa Fe, New Mexico 87501. *email: onenessmailbox@yahoo.com.*